Living Well with Food Intolerance

His Tame

It can look and act like
— but it's NO allergy

Treat the Cause.
Stop the Symptoms.
Get Your Life Back Today!

BY MARCUS LAUX, N.D.

Disclaimer: The material in this presentation is for informational purposes only and not intended for the treatment or diagnosis of individual disease. Please visit a qualified medical or other health professional for specifically diagnosing any ailments mentioned or discussed in detail in this material.

ISBN: 978-1-893910-66-9
Printed in the United States
Freedom Press
1861 N. Topanga Cyn Blvd.
Topanga, CA 90290
Bulk Orders Available: (800) 959-9797
E-mail: info@freedompressonline.com

Living Well with Food Intolerance
by Dr. Marcus Laux, co-author and editor,
with Dr. Grace Abbot, Dr. Camille Lieners, Dr. Isabella Mayer,
Dr. Albert Missbichler, Dr. Markus Pfisterer and Mag. Helmut Schmutz

❧ CONTENTS ❧

Introduction

Histamine intolerance. A hidden epidemic is finally revealed. This condition, which can cause food intolerance—often incorrectly labeled as a food allergy—is experienced widely by too many, yet is virtually unknown. Now, an emerging field of research with great promise has arrived in North America. For those of you coping with food intolerance symptoms, but who have not been able to fully connect them to your diet, you are going to find an effective natural solution; indeed, a true cure is possible.

One of the foremost reasons for writing this book was to help people struggling from histamine intolerance be aware of the fact that they are by no means alone and that now, for the first time, there are effective and natural means to resolving this problem.

The authors of this book have written a simple story to allow persons suffering from histamine intolerance to seek their own answers and find natural solutions for themselves. We want to empower those folks to help themselves.

The purpose of this book is to help everyone suffering from histamine intolerance to orient themselves to the diagnosis of their condition and become aware of encouraging new science and effective treatment options.

Healing is possible with Mother Nature. In the case of histamine intolerance, technology in the service of nature is used to deliver the exact natural agent to target the problem and heal the discomfort of histamine intolerance.

You have taken a significant and meaningful step with us towards understanding this disease, which is regrettably on the increase worldwide.

This book is your start to a full recovery. It is closer than ever and it can be a much smoother and comfortable path with the new research and natural solutions revealed in these pages. Here's to hope and healing for all of us. It is in our hands and in our control. That is the good news, and an amazing opportunity for our best health ever. Here's to your being naturally well today, and every day.   — Marcus Laux, N.D.

1. Is It Food Allergy or Food Intolerance?

With certain foods have you ever thought that you have a true love-hate relationship?

Do you love pizza, red wine, hot dogs, and ham and pastrami? Have you ever enjoyed a Reuben sandwich at a deli? How about Gouda, parmesan, cheddar and Swiss cheese? Tuna, mackerel, or smoked herring? Papaya, tomatoes, bananas, avocados, sauerkraut or spinach salad might also be some of your favorites.

But do you *hate* the way you feel after enjoying these foods?

Today, millions of people are finally learning that their irritable bowel syndrome (especially stomach upset, cramping, flatulence and diarrhea), migraine headaches, sinus problems, asthma-like reactions, and skin eruptions, to name a few of the most prominent symptoms, that any of these could well be the result of eating these foods. We love them. We can't escape them. We sometimes even eat them without thinking or consciously knowing what we are doing at that moment! But our bodies hate them. All of these foods are rich in histamine, an inflammatory substance doctors and scientists are only now coming to grips with when it comes to your health. The condition is known as histamine intolerance or HIT. And if your health is taking a HIT with any of these symptoms, you might well be a victim.

But if you're suffering these symptoms, you don't need to despair that you will always be the victim of such a love-hate food relationship. There's hope on the horizon—and it couldn't come too soon for millions of people who have been victimized by food intolerance.

Since at least the 1980s, doctors and medical specialists throughout the world have been making diligent attempts to gain the widespread acceptance of a new disease classification: food intolerance.

The diagnosis and medical recognition of this condition were, indeed, quite complicated because the symptoms such as rhinitis, headaches, skin rashes, and gastrointestinal disorders are manifested in the presence of many other diseases as well.

Nevertheless and undeterred, the doctors concerned with this subject persisted in their efforts to investigate the underlying cause and possible connections of these often seemingly unrelated symptoms directly to a person's diet.

Initially, the conventional medical wisdom was to assume that these reactions and symptoms were merely additional forms of known food allergies. Allergies are caused by immune overreactions and the production of substances in the blood known as antibodies and immunoglobulins with names like IgE and IgG. We test for these markers when trying to sleuth out food allergies. Officially, some eight foods are considered to be allergens and account for 90 percent of the reactions (which, in extreme cases of anaphylactic shock, can include death). These include dairy, egg, peanuts, tree nuts, shellfish, fish, soy and wheat. However, when this group of individuals was tested, no immune reactions were identified! The tests simply yielded no positive results. The researchers found no immune response, which would indicate a true allergic reaction.

Over time, this logical first assumption was growing ever more doubtful and appeared flatly incorrect.

Well, if not an allergy after all, then what was causing the symptoms?

When the patients were questioned further to dig deeper into this unfolding mystery, doctors discovered that they experienced several of their symptoms together after the ingestion of various foods. However, the follow-up laboratory investigations performed on these individual foods still revealed none were caused by IgE-related allergic reactions or corresponding IgG antibodies. Therefore, researchers had to look for other causes in individuals affected by these perplexing and persistent unexplained conditions.

To add to this evolving mystery, the foods that were suspected of creating the various symptoms did not appear to be related. At least at first glance, so read on.

A large number of food categories and individual items were under investigation: seafood such as tuna; prepared foods such as sauerkraut; alcoholic beverages including champagne, red wine but not white; fruits and vegetables such as tomatoes and bananas and some cheeses but not others, to name but a few of the foods that seemed to be causing the symptoms, so finding a common thread seemed at best remote.

At that time, there were no specific diagnostic procedures to identify food intolerance. All doctors could do was establish a "working diagnosis by exclusion" of all other possibilities, if they wished to risk labeling their patients with the still highly controversial condition offered up by a few medical mavericks in the field.

In 2003-2004, however, research with which my co-authors were closely involved delivered a ground-breaking development. At last, the definitive clinical and chemical procedures to demonstrate the link between all of these foods became available.

Yes, it finally became possible to establish an accurate and the definitive diagnosis of histamine-related food intolerance, and declare it as one of the major food intolerance categories. This clinically validated procedure led to the acceptance of histamine intolerance as a distinct disease entity in medical circles.

This breakthrough also heralded in more exacting research focused on this disease process—which can be highly unpleasant for any person suffering from it—as well as set the goal line for successful management and treatment of this growing global disease with satifying success rates.

Indeed, the discovery of this link and the keys to successfully managing this form of food intolerance will be thoroughly discussed throughout the rest of this book. Our goal is to provide reliable medical, nutritional, and lifestyle support and understanding for the millions of people who are affected, and for all the medical professionals who will be called upon to help them. We will present the causes of histamine intolerance, ways to self diagnosis your condition and as well as diagnose clinically, and the most effective, proven solutions to manage, maintain, and take back control in your life.

2. Histamine—The Good, The Bad, and The Ugly

What is histamine? And why does it cause such a ruckus in the world of dieticians, gastroenterologists, allergists, dermatologists, and among millions of patients with uncomfortable systemic complaints, whether digestive symptoms, migraines, skin eruptions, and/or other discomforting symptoms? Well, histamine has been known for nearly a century. It is a biogenic amine (messenger substance that combines with other molecules) like tyramines, cadaverines, putrescines that all can trigger allergy-like reactions. But these aren't allergies! Indeed, such incorrect diagnoses in the past and present have led to unnecessary suffering for those affected.

Research into histamine was started in 1907 when it was first synthesized by the German chemists A. Windaus and W. Vogt. Just three years later (1910), Henry H. Dale and P. P. Laidlaw discovered that histamine is an endogenous substance, and they described a few basic functions of histamine. Histamine is a natural substance that acts as a "tissue hormone" and a "neurotransmitter" in humans as well as in animals. In any living organism, histamine plays an important role in allergic reactions and is involved in defending the body from foreign substances via supporting the immune system.

Histamine is important for our well-being and proper functioning as well, with a dynamic balance the key. It performs important functions in the body but is also a powerful inflammatory vasodilator with many toxic effects when levels are high. Our foods are made up of many naturally occurring compounds and they have varying effects on us. For literally millions of us, we have an inadequate production or reserve of the necessary enzyme needed to break down histamine from some of these food sources. Much like lactose intolerance that benefits from the lactase enzyme to break down milk sugars, histamine intolerance is caused by inadequate amounts of diamine oxidase (DAO). DAO should be naturally present in our digestive system, but when missing, or in too little amounts, histame ingestion can lead to very uncomfortable systems.

One of the main effects of histamine found in the body's tissues and throughout our circulatory system in our blood is to serve as a stimulating neurotransmitter. It is pro-inflammatory, meaning it can set into motion many of the unpleasant symptoms characteristic of food intolerance.

Histamine is a very active *mediator* (messenger substance) for a large number of biochemical reactions and, as such, it is highly modulated and regulated by various body systems just to keep it in check and balanced.

Histamine is the foremost representative of a class of substances collectively known as "biogenic amines. These include a number of largely aliphatic polyamines, which occur as natural metabolic products in nearly all living organisms. In addition to histamine, other well known members of this class of substances include serotonin, and spermidine, among the others mentioned earlier.

Until recently, relatively little was known about the diverse biological functions of these organic compounds. Recent research has shown that polyamines possess essential regulatory properties in respect to cellular growth and division (mitosis). Furthermore, even at very low concentrations they are extremely reactive mediators of a number of metabolic processes, which are yet to be fully delineated through research.

In nerve cells (neurons) and other cells that can be stimulated, polyamines serve as neurotransmitters (among other functions). As neurotransmitters, they play an essential role in the regulation of synaptic activity, nerve transmission, and cellular regeneration.

Biochemically speaking, this biogenic amine is produced from the transformation of the amino acid histidine and is primarily stored in white blood cells called granulocytes and mast cells in our respiratory, gastrointestinal and other tissues.

So the question now is, how does histamine benefit us? Well, let's take an insect bite, like from a mosquito looking for a meal or when a wasp stings in its defense. Their venom causes immediate histamine to be released from our mast cells, which lie below the uppermost layers of skin. This histamine is the molecular messenger, so to speak, which informs the nerve cells through its receptors that something is wrong and needs attention.

Bee and wasp venom also contain some histamine itself, which enhances the victim's perception of pain.

Only when this histamine messenger has delivered its attention/stimulatory message, does the nerve cell sound the alarm, which then triggers a cascade of escalating reactions. This concert of cascading reactions starts with the perception of pain and end with swelling, circulatory changes, reddening of the skin, and itching.

This trigger mechanism is, in principle, always the same, independent of the actual cause of the irritation initiation. In other words, independent of whether the person has been bitten by a mosquito or horsefly, or stung by a honey bee or wolf wasp, bitten by sea nettle or a man-o-war tentacle, or simply pricked by plant stinging nettle—the process is the same.

Regardless of whether you are sensitive or reactive to the above list or other potential environmental factors, histamine is always the substance that delivers the actual message.

Histamine is an important mediator in other ways as well. For example, in the gastrointestinal tract, histamine is critical to the regulation of gastric acid production, gastrointestinal motility, and also to the regulation of the sleeping-waking circadian rhythm of the central nervous system. It even plays a role in control of appetite (yes, controlling histamine can probably help weight loss, too).

The Real Culprit: Sources of Histamine in the Diet

I've mentioned that histamine is produced by the body. But that's not the only source of histamine—and here's where your diet plays a critical role.

We now know that histamine is found at high levels in some foods and at even higher levels in many prepared and packaged foods.

This brings us to the actual and central "culprit" in persons who suffer from food intolerance.

We are dealing here with the histamine found in substances from outside the body, particularly coming in from foods; this form of histamine is generally consumed and absorbed by the body.

Histamine is formed in several ways, and often in combination with each other. It can be formed by fermentation, or storage over a longer period of time, and through various production processes. The fact is that a surprising number of foods contain this active substance, some in considerable quantities. Higher histamine content is capable of causing significant discomfort and unpleasant reactions if it is not degraded rapidly and efficiently by normal enzymatic action within the organism, as it is naturally equipped to do so on demand. If degraded or digested, then there is no reaction, no symptoms, except tasty food!

Histamine ingested with food is degraded within the body by the aid of DAO produced on site by the intestinal mucosa. The exact amount of enzyme production, its availability, and the extent of enzymatic degradation differs greatly from person to person, as we are unique and live different lifestyles.

Symptoms

Sensitive individuals can show their reaction to biogenic amines that have not been degraded by an increase in pulse rate, a sensation of warmth and flushing, whereas the ingestion of large quantities can lead to a fever, vomiting, reddening of the skin, itching, rash, and much more.

How Histamine is Metabolized

The digestive system is a collective term for all the organs involved in our inner food processing plant. From our mouth, tongue, and teeth, to our stomach, pancreas, and liver, to our intestines, appendix, to anus; we indeed, have an amazingly sophisticated and synchronized gastrointestinal system, or GI tract. In essence, its job is to take foreign substances and and turn what is useable into us-our flesh, blood, and bone. It has to break down, digest, absorb, and transport valuable nutrients into the body, while managing our inner immune border patrol and eliminate the wastes efficiently and regularly.

The main functions of the intestines are to absorb the utilizable nutrient parts of foods and eliminate the indigestible and undesirable components of our food.

However, digestion itself is defined as the absorption of food with the help of enzymes. In this field of research, histamine intolerance has been mainly focused on the small intestines because this is the main site of dynamic digestion and most absorption of the nutrient constituents from our food (carbohydrates, proteins, fat, vitamins, salt and water). This is the place where the histamine ingested with food is processed. This is also the place where DAO—this critically important enzyme for the degradation of histamine—is produced.

Renowned allergist Reinhart Jarisch, M.D., of Austria, was one of the global researchers who had discovered that certain food reactions were not inciting an actual immune reaction in his patients, and therefore the reaction was not a classic allergy. The trick was to find out what was going on.

Dr. Jarisch enlisted the help of experts in food allergy and food intolerance diagnostic testing who discovered that many of the patients lacked adequate activity of an enzyme called diamine oxidase (DAO). This enzyme is specific and necessary to digest histamine.

And once these people began eliminating certain foods from their diets such as red wine, cured meats, and tomatoes, they began to improve greatly.

In the population around three percent of people have significantly low DAO activity in their blood and about 25 percent have highly reduced DAO activity, according to Dr. Jarisch and his co-researchers, based on extrapolations from clinical, experimental, and epidemiological research.

The causes of reduced activity are multi-factorial and probably include some genetic but mainly environmental factors. For example, one potent DAO inhibitor is alcohol. Couple that with the fact that some alcoholic beverages like red wine are high in histamine anyway, and it could be sure set up for problems for suspectible folks!

The most important regulator of histamine found in our tissues and in blood circulation is the endogenous enzyme known as diamine oxidase.

Depending on the current needs of the organism, this enzyme converts the histamine present into imidazole acetaldehyde. Importantly, imidazole acetaldehyde is a substance that causes no negative effect in our body. The diamine oxidase enzyme inactivates the histamine directly and converts it into a nonactive metabolite. It's the end of the line for that histamine.

Through this mechanism, histamine levels are kept in constant check and dynamically balanced.

Thus, the perfectly controlled histamine levels required to achieve metabolic balance between the many biochemical reactions necessary to deal with the body's daily needs is ensured for our vital health, while, simultaneously, potentially harmful excessive levels of histamine are effectively avoided by efficient DAO enzyme degradation.

But what if we don't produce enough DAO? Actually, tens of millions of people globally do not. Any imbalance in the required quantity or activity of the DAO enzyme, caused by any number of different factors, may lead to the various symptoms of histamine intolerance. Much like people who do not produce or produce too little of the lactase enzyme necessary to digest dairy foods, people lacking DAO also suffer unnecessarily. Now there is a way to treat the cause, stop the symptoms and get your life back!

3. How to Diagnose Histamine Intolerance

oo many people worldwide suffer from the symptoms of histamine intolerance without even being aware of the cause. They can go through an endless odyssey of visits to doctors' offices and specialty clinics, without receiving a correct diagnosis or getting any lasting symptom improvement. Unfortunately, far too often the cause of their symptoms is never identified and their complaints are attributed to other diseases, or just written off as being psychosomatic. With subsequent medical visits, if negative allergy tests results are returned, again, the person's symptoms may get symptomatic drug treatment with the diagnosis usually assigned to the category of psychosomatic ailments, or idiopathic etiology—which means cause unknown. There is now a better way. There is a much brighter future awaiting you.

Food Allergy or Food Intolerance

In order to understand the causes and effects of histamine intolerance it is essential to first make the distinction between intolerance and allergy. This is because the two entities tend to be spoken of interchangeably and/or confused for each other too often. They are not the same. But, because of the similarity of symptoms in the two diseases, even though the medical and biochemical demarcation is quite clear and categorically distinct, they get lumped together. We now set the record straight, and in doing so, help establish an end to this once cryptic epidemic.

While they both can be classified as adverse reactions to foods with similar, and even exact symptoms possible, the mechanism of causation is completely different. Often, time of occurrence is vastly different too.

Allergy

An allergy stems from the immune system and usually happens within a few minutes of eating certain foods. These offending foods are generally divided into eight groups. A food allergy is a quickly appearing excessive or over-reaction of the body to specific substances also known as allergens) in the environment.

The actual function of the immune system is to protect the body from bacteria, viruses, cancer cells and foreign substances. In cases of allergic reactions, our defense system over responds to its intended goal, as it essentially has an abnormal reaction to a normal substance.

In cases of allergy, the immune system is activated by substances that cause no reaction in a healthy (or non-allergic or -sensitive individual) body. These substances (known as allergens) may be inhaled (e.g. house dust, pollen) or ingested with food (e.g., shellfish, nuts). If an allergen is found as a component in the food, then this condition is referred to as a food allergy.

However, the course of an allergic reaction is essentially and significantly different from the course of food intolerance.

The allergen is ingested with food and identified by the immune system through antibodies and immunoglobulins with certain members of the alphabet attached to their name. In allergies, this occurs in most cases through antibodies of the IgE type. These antibodies can be found on the surfaces of the respiratory system's mast cells and can activate, if immunologically stimulated by the allergen being recognized by it. Large quantities of histamine are stored in mast cells, and can be released when triggered this way, and the alert and alarm allergy process is now full steam ahead!

The histamine that is rapidly released leads to acute symptoms, such as sneezing, diarrhea, skin rash, and more, by activating other cells and tissues throughout the body and promoting blood circulation in those affected tissues.

In principle, any food is potentially capable of causing allergies. The most common allergies are those to crustaceans or shellfish, milk, fish, soybean, wheat, eggs, nuts and various types of vegetables and fruits.

The symptoms may differ, depending on the intensity of the allergy or the allergen content of food. They include the following:

* Swollen lips and a swollen face
* A tingling sensation in the oral cavity and lips
* Vomiting, cramps and/or spasms in the stomach, diarrhea
* A sudden runny/or congested nose
* Swelling of the larynx, asthma, breathlessness
* Itching skin, rash, swelling
* Drop in blood pressure

In the worst case scenario, an allergic reaction can lead to anaphylactic shock. This condition is characterized by a dramatically excessive immune reaction which may lead to the patient's death in minutes.

Once someone has been sensitized to an allergen, every subsequent contact with that allergen is immediately identified and processed by the immune system from its impeccable archives.

The complete process of an allergic reaction has still not been fully elucidated to date. There are still many questions, for example as to how environmental factors (chemical substances) as well as genetic factors (heredity) play their role. But what we do know that true food allergy reactions in general are rather immediate and involve the body mounting an unnecessary immune response.

Food intolerance

In contrast to food allergy, food intolerance does not involve the immune system. Thus, there is no allergen identified, no antibody response, and no histamine released by immune cells. But histamine still does plays a BIG role. This time though the histamine is released from foods!

The various food intolerances are usually associated with an enzyme deficiency or the inhibition of an enzyme's activity that is responsible for the degradation of that specific food component, whether its an enzyme needed for lactose, gluten, or histamine, in the body.

If these food constituents are not adequately degraded, then this process can lead to undesired reactions. Food intolerance can be considered a matter of an enzyme issue, whether from deficiency, defect, or inhibition.

For example, lactose intolerance is a common type of food intolerance. Individuals suffering from lactose intolerance suffer from a deficiency of the enzyme lactase and are unable or poorly digest lactose, a type of sugar contained in milk. The principal symptom is discomfort and diarrhea in nearly all cases, which may occur 15 to 30 minutes after the consumption of lactose; the second major symptom is flatulence. Further symptoms may be a rumbling stomach, intestinal gases, nausea after meals and abdominal cramps.

Usually the symptoms of this class of food intolerance are confined to the gastrointestinal tract. However, histamine intolerance is an exception to this rule.

Histaminosis or histamine intolerance is a term used to denote the intolerance of high histamine-containing foods or the inability of the human body to degrade the ingested histamine in adequate quantities. Due to poor functioning or a deficiency of the enzyme diamine oxidase, a person is unable to degrade the histamine ingested with their food.

Thus, histamine is able to cross the intestinal barrier—largely unimpeded and unaltered—and may cause the same symptoms in the body as those that occur when histamine is released from mast cells in response to allergic reactions.

Larger quantities of histamine lead to acute symptoms such as breathlessness, a drop in blood pressure, reddening of the skin, skin flushing, itching and/or rash, nausea, vomiting, headache and diarrhea.

As food intolerance causes the same allergy-like symptoms, it is very commonly and incorrectly mistaken for a food allergy event.

However, allergy testing can neither discover nor demonstrate a classical IgE response. Therefore, in the past, food intolerance used to be incorrectly named a "pseudoallergy."

A diamine oxidase deficiency may be congenital or acquired.

Today, there is insufficient data regarding the prevalence of a genetic enzyme defect in the general population. But we do have reason to believe that our diets are far higher in histamine than ever before because of all the processed foods which tend to have histamine librators, DAO inhibitors and frequently elevated histamine levels. That is why an acquired histamine intolerance is probably the most likely widespread causation of this condition, for many known reasons.

One recognized common cause of active inhibition is frequently due to the intake of medications. From taking drugs, a person suffers from excessively low diamine oxidase activity caused by the drug's active inhibition of this valuable enzyme.

Many drugs, in fact, are active inhibiting substances, including painkillers, asthma medications, expectorants, blood pressure-reducing medications, and antibiotics; all are known to inhibit the activity of enzymes. Alcohol is well known to be an inhibitor of diamine oxidase as well (as they share the exact same enzyme needed to be processed).

DAO-inhibiting Drugs

Active Agent	Application
Acetylcysteine	Cough
Ambroxol	Cough
Aminophylline	Asthma
Amitriptyline	Antidepressant
Chloroquine	Malaria
Clavulanic acid	Antibiotic
Isoniazid	Antibiotic
Metamizole	Pain
Metoclopramide	Nausea
Propafenone	Cardiac arrhythmia
Verapamil	Cardiovascular disease

nd, if that is not enough, there are other concerns in relation to histamine exposure. Histamine intolerance may also be caused by foods that do not contain histamine itself, but do contain substances that "release" or "liberate" histamine from the endogenous mast cells without the assistance of IgE antibodies.

Histamine Intolerance's Symptoms

Individuals who suffer from histamine intolerance often experience the symptoms listed below. These symptoms may vary significantly in terms of severity and frequency.

Many patients have several symptoms such as migraine headaches with flushing and fatigue, whereas others may experience one or two of those mentioned below, in their own unique combination including:

* Abdominal pain, spasms
* Diarrhea, with alternating normal phases ("irritable colon")
* Chronic constipation
* Flatulence and a sensation of fullness, often *very massive* and independent of meals, occasionally when waking up in the morning
* Headache, frequently migraine-like and *therapy resistant*
* A runny nose, watering eyes, usually during or after meals, without known allergies
* Skin rash, eczema, nettle rash, partly of long duration, partly sporadic and without an identifiable cause
* Rosacea-like skin rash of the face
* Attacks of dizziness, frequently a sensation of "cotton wool in the head"
* Sudden changes in psychic states(e.g., aggressiveness, lack of attention, poor concentration, lack of focus, etc), often during or after a meal
* "Extreme exhaustion" usually during or after a meal, leading to a compulsive urge to sleep and requiring several hours of sleep in many cases. Quite often the person does not awake refreshed, but feels completely spent.
* Chills, shivers, discomfort, low blood pressure (rarely high blood pressure)
* Intolerance noted to certain foods (see list in the appendix).

A person might experience the above mentioned unexplained symptoms for several years. In some patients the symptoms may occur occasionally or even suddenly, "out of the blue," but often reported to have started after a previous gastrointestinal compromise, whether infection, disease or operation.

The many symptoms that can emanate from histamine-mediated reactions in the body were captured in the following chart from The American Society for Nutrition's prestigious *American Journal of Clinical Nutrition*.

Summary of histamine-mediated symptoms

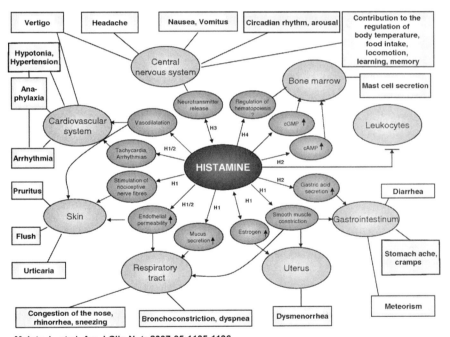

Maintz, L. et al. Am J Clin Nutr 2007;85:1185-1196

In addition to histamine intolerance, some people report suffering from other food intolerances as well.

These include becoming sensitized to other foods (gluten) plus additional other enzyme deficiency symptoms, especially related to sugars such as lactose or fructose. Therefore, an exact documentation of the patient's medical history as well as a documentation of the intolerant foods, and targeted diagnosis, are particularly important in order to offer comprehensive guidance and therapy.

Forms of Diagnosis

With all the advances in modern medicine, it is regrettable that until recently histamine intolerance was just another one of many ambiguous health concerns. Even still, many medical specialists are not yet aware of the most recent research advances that can improve lives fast.

Fortunately, since 2003 we have a laboratory test that allows identification of histamine intolerance in many of these patients. This makes it possible to establish a specific diagnosis now, which then can be treated definitively and effectively. What a terrific advance in medicine, for doctors in clinical practice, and people everywhere who knew they had a problem, but with no credible help in sight! Your doctor can now evaluate tests for DAO enzyme activity and histamine levels.

A combination of different methods is needed to make a reliable diagnosis. These include the following:

* Differential diagnosis: Exclusion of diseases that cause similar symptoms.
* Blood test: Measurement of DAO enzyme activity.
* Elimination diet: All foods rich in histamine and all histamine-releasing food and medications are avoided for a trial period of time (four weeks).

In the differential diagnosis it is important to exclude organic diseases, as well as intolerance of lactose or fructose because many individuals with histamine intolerance suffer from several other food intolerances as well.

Recent procedures to demonstrate histamine intolerance are increasingly accurate and provide exacting information about this process and your condition.

In particular, the measurement of histamine levels in conjunction with the measurement of DAO activity is currently the most reliable and commonly used method to demonstrate the condition.

The elimination diet can be used too. Its drawback is that all substances containing histamine or releasing histamine have not yet been accurately determined. This is especially true for prepared foods.

Thus, inaccurate results or false results may be obtained. Besides, one should bear in mind the fact that foods today are composed of the most diverse combinations of substances, which renders a true elimination diet nearly impossible.

Depending on the treating doctor's experience, a combination of the above mentioned diagnostic procedures is most likely the best means of achieving the goal of identifying yourself as experiencing histamine intolerance. Once you know you have it, though, there's some good news. You can become symptom-free. And yes, you can be cured. Even at very least, feel like it, as you have your life back, without pain and suffering.

4. The Natural Solution: A Low-histamine Diet with Supplemental Diamine Oxidase (DAO)

Once histamine intolerance has been diagnosed with certainty, the person will definitely want to follow specific dietary recommendations. The number of clinics specializing in this is slowly growing, but the patient is usually left to his own means as far as understanding food intolerance and adjusting his or her lifestyle to the challenges of daily living with this condition.

However, seeking out the assistance a skilled specialist in allergies, dietary planning, and natural medicine is recommended whenever feasible, for ensuring best health outcomes.

Dietary recommendations for a low-histamine diet

In cases of histamine intolerance it is advisable to adopt and maintain a low-histamine diet.

Avoidance of histamine-containing food and beverages is a basic prerequisite. Histamine cannot be destroyed by common methods of cooking such as freezing, boiling, baking or microwave heating. Histamine is both heat-stable and cold-stable. It is unfortunate, but while vitamins and minerals can diminish from food storage and preparation, not so for the histamine.

People with histamine intolerance will benefit substantially by knowing which food products contain histamine and might lead to their undesired symptoms. Interestingly, offending foods might not seem much related.

But you can be sure that cured meats such as pastrami and cold cuts, aged cheeses, and smoked fish are among the commonest culprits.

This list is headed-up by red wine, champagne, aged cheese, salami, fish and sauerkraut, as their measurements have shown the highest histamine content in them.

However, there is a large variation and differences noted between even similar products, primarily due to the degree of freshness and/or the maturation (the aging or fermentation) process of these food products.

The histamine content of some common foods is listed in the table below. This list is a small representation of all histamine containing food products available. Notably, individual products of certain food categories differ drastically from others; this again is indicative of the fact that the causal factor is the type of fermentation rather than the histamine content of the basic product.

Histamine content of foods and beverages

FOOD	NAME	HISTAMINE [mg/l or mg/kg]
Red wine	Rotwein Nickelsdorf	0, 05
	St.Laurent 2004	11
	Syrah Südafrika 2004	0, 05
	Merlot 2001	1, 25
	Zweigelt 2002	3
White wine	Chardonnay	0, 15
	Sauvignon Blanc Beerenauslese	0, 05
	Sämling 88 Jungfernlese 2004	0, 1
Sparkling wine	Spumanti Martini Asti	0
Beer	Wheat beer	0
	Unfiltered beer	0
Vinegar	Red wine vinegar	0,1
	Balsamico	1, 5
Sauces	Fish sauce	490
	Soy sauce dark	1, 05
	Soy sauce	0, 9
	Teriyaki marinade	0, 75

Sauerkraut	Sauerkraut	130
Meat	Garlic salami	0, 25
	Herbage salami	230
	Prosciutto	0
	Haussalami	0, 25
	Kantwurst	4, 5
Cheese	Soft cheese	0, 6
	Bergkäse	500
	Turkish feta cheese	14
	Raclette cheese	1
	Emmentaler	40, 5
	Grated pizza cheese	0, 75
	Camembert	0
	Blue veined cheese	11
	Geheimratskäse	0, 25
Fish	Tuna	0, 75
	Catfish	2
	Smoked salmon	0
	Salmon / stored 1 week at 4°C	135
	Tuna / stored 4 weeks at 4°C	300
Tomato	Fresh tomato	4
	Ketchup	4
Spinach	Spinach leaves frozen	12
Chocolate	Dark chocolate	0
Fruit	Carrot juice fresh	0
	Strawberry	0
	Apple	0
	Kiwi	0
	Banana	2, 5
Nuts	Cashews	0
Yeast	Yeast	0, 5

The basic rule is to remember: the longer a food is stored or left to mature, the greater its histamine content.

Fresh meat contains no or very little histamine. However, when meat is processed further, the maturation process results in the accumulation of biogenic amines.

The same is true for fish. Fresh fish contains no or very little histamine. However, fish spoils very easily and this leads to a rapid accumulation of histamine due to bacteria. Further processing, which includes salting, smoke-drying, marinating and preservation, may increase the histamine content. Hazardously high histamine concentrations may develop in specific types of fish which are rich in histidine, such as

* Tuna fish
* Mackerel
* Sardines

In addition to foods rich in histamine, some substances by themselves do not contain large quantities of histamine but stimulate the release of endogenous histamine (histamine liberators).

These include chocolate (cocoa), tomatoes, strawberries, citrus fruits, pineapple, papaya, mango, buckwheat, crustaceans and shellfish, nuts (especially nuts that are old or rancid or were handled poorly during processing and handling), sunflower seeds, vinegar and mustard.

Additives in food may also act as histamine liberators, such as glutamate, benzoate, colorants, sulfites and nitrites. Take heed and pay close attention!

Nitrite preservatives in cured meats are a real problem. So is monosodium glutamate or MSG in foods. Avoid these at all costs! Check labels twice!

Foods or medications that exert a negative effect on the activity of the enzyme diamine oxidase constitute another important group. The most important food constituent of this type is alcohol, whose degradation product acetaldehyde is a very effective inhibitor of DAO.

A well-established dietary supplement that may act as DAO inhibitor is acetyl cysteine (NAC), and a drug example is ambroxol.

Foods to Avoid

Fish (<0.1 – 13000 mg/kg)

The following should be avoided:

* Tuna fish, mackerel, sardines, anchovy, all shellfish, herring
* Particularly in preserved form, or marinated, salted or dried fish
* Smoked fish
* Rolled pickled herring
* Fish sauces

Fish and seafood are particularly susceptible to microbial spoilage, which causes large quantities of histamine to be formed. Under proper processing and storage however, deep-frozen seafood and preserved fish is hardly affected. Adding salt and/or smoke-drying, however, may increase the histamine content of preserved fish. Marinated fish might contain histamine due to being marinated in vinegar.

Your best bet is to consume either fresh or deep frozen fish.

Meat (< 0.1 – 318 mg/kg)

Fresh or deep-frozen meat and poultry are best choices.

* Avoid all processed, smoke-dried and pickled sausages, salami, bacon, ham, smoked meats.
* Avoid preserved and processed meat products in general, and never heat them up.
* When buying any cut, sliced, or ground meats, make sure they are super fresh, eat promptly, and avoid long storage times.
* Ensure that all animal products are adequately packaged, re-sealed after use promptly, and continuously well-chilled under constant refrigeration.

Cheese (< 0.1 – 555 mg/kg)

Note the following with regard to cheese:

* Largely free of histamine: cottage cheese and other types of fresh cheese
* Cheeses like Tilsiter, butter cheese or young Gouda contain very low concentrations of histamine.

* Caution is advised in cases of cheeses that take a long time to mature. The longer the maturation or aged period, the greater is the histamine content. This is particularly true for hard cheeses like Emmentaler, Bergkäse and parmesan.
* In cases of soft and blue cheeses one should avoid mature and overripe pieces.
* Cheeses produced from raw milk contain more histamine than cheese made from pasteurized milk because of the flora growth present in the raw milk.

For low histamine content, select fresh cottage cheese, milk, yogurt and cream.

Bread and confectionery

Individuals with a histamine deficiency are usually unable to tolerate bread and confectionery. The reason is the use of yeast—which contains a large quantity of histamine—and other raising agents.

Please note the following:
* Yeast is used for baking, for production of wine and beer, and in the food industry.
* Yeast as well as chemical raising agents and baking powder are very rich in histamine.
* Eliminating bread and confectionery completely from one's diet is neither feasible nor fun.
* However, it would be advisable to avoid cake, confectionery and sweets that contain large quantities of raising agents.
* Alternatives: yeast-free confections and breads are becoming more available in stores.

Vegetables

The following types of vegetables should be avoided:
* Sauerkraut, spinach, tomatoes, eggplant, avocado, mushrooms
* Commercially prepared salads

* It should be noted that marinated foods can also contain histamine because of the histamine content of vinegar.

All other types of vegetables may be consumed, provided they are either fresh or deep-frozen.

Alcohol

Histamine is contained in wine in an alcoholic solution. Therefore, wine is tolerated even more poorly than other histamine-containing foods.

Alcohol also inhibits the enzyme DAO, which is responsible for the degradation of histamine. This is a double dose of discomfort for those sensitive folks!

The majority of persons with histamine intolerance are dependent on maintaining a low-histamine to even histamine-free diets in order to avoid bouts of intolerance. With perseverance, please know it is possible to achieve appreciable improvements and symptom relief for most of us.

However, in reality, histamine-rich foods can sneak into our diets at any time due to the composition of prepared food products and undeclared additives in even seemingly safe foods, as well as due to food storage and handling. There is another important protective step for you to take.

Diamine Oxidase Supplements: Proven Safe and Effective

Today, for your strategic health advantage is the all-natural DAO nutritional supplement (e.g., Histame). Clinically studied in Europe and proven to work, Histame is available for the first time ever in North America.

You may not be able to always avoid hidden histamine or dodge its unwanted effects solely through dietary deletions and lifestyle changes, but you can always remember to halt any histamine havoc by being prepared with supplemental DAO enzymes. Your health and your comfort can now take advantage of the most naturally talented and nutritionally targeted ally in your food fight and win!

Just as the enzyme lactase is taken as a supportive measure in cases of lactose intolerance, a high-quality DAO supplement can support your natural balance for those wanting to tame histamine intolerance. It is interesting to note that histamine intolerance could be referred to as histaminosis—too much histamine. Now also consider another common reference name for DAO, referred to as "histaminase"—the specific enzyme that degrades histamine.

Supplementing with this specific DAO enzyme supplement before any suspect meal in concert with a prudent menu make-over can lead to a remarkable and reliable improvement in your overall enjoyment and quality of life.

One amazing advantage in taking the DAO enzyme is its real-time activity, its immediate efficacy that can be felt in terms of your comfort and relief of symptoms. This all-natural DAO supplement works fast, indeed very fast, when you want relief the most. People with HIT have reported immediate favorable responses with symptom relief after taking the DAO enzyme supplement.

You do not need to take DAO for several weeks or months in order to experience any improvement. It can literally happen in minutes into a meal. Truly remarkable health benefits you can judge for yourself from a simple natural solution. Targeted and proven, safe and effective. I'm so glad to share this breaking research with you. It will be life-changing, and it is so simple now that we understand this condition better. Nature has the best answer.

For your consideration as well, it has been observed that people who have become symptom-free for a long period of time by following this protocol, and with DAO supplementation and then suddenly revert back to consuming lots of high histamine-containing foods, can and often do have their symptoms flair up.

Even with the additional intake of DAO enzymes, it appears not to be able to compensate for such over-indulgences, which could then lead to undesirable reactions once again.

But, in this regards, there really is good news to share. Your life can improve enormously and without having to be forever on guard. Many people report that when they consume moderate histamine levels only in their diet and regularly take their supplemental DAO enzymes, they have been able to maintain their comfort and stay symptom free.

You can create and control your health destiny. I highly encourage all of us to do this for ourselves. You can be free from discomfort and limitation. You have the power to manifest your unique body balance through making smart health decisions and living them! It has been said, it's not the years of life, but the life in your years that counts most dearly. DAO is a simple enzyme that can change your life. DAO is a natural solution for millions of folks who have suffered without a known cause, without effective therapy, until now.

Appendixes: Case Reports

I n clinical practice one is frequently confronted with patients who complain of chronic symptoms such as headaches, gastrointestinal discomforts, abnormal blood pressure, poor liver detoxification, etc. for several years.

In many of these cases, conventional medicine has very little if anything of value to offer. Doctors frequently prescribe medications that promise alleviation of the symptoms but achieve this end in very few cases.

Apart from a mild and transient abatement of symptoms these therapies do not bring about any cure.

Enormous advances have been made in acute medical crisis with technology, but when it comes to helping chronic diseases, this is still the healing realm of natural medicine where it leads the way to the future.

Case report I

Patient: Male, early forties, complains of recurrent headache for several years, occasional migraine, chronic fatigue and changes of mood. In fact, he had resigned to his condition because he had been experiencing these complaints for more than 20 years. He always kept his headache medicine on him.

Neurologically the patient was normal. Various imaging procedures showed no abnormalities. No deviations from the normal condition were observed in respect to hormones. The patient's mild postural disorder was treated by an osteopath. Acupuncture also failed to improve his condition. All measures available to conventional medicine had been used to investigate the patient's condition and no cause had been found. One symptom he had is worthy of note; the fact that this patient complained of regular and significant flatulence.

The patient's digestive capacity and intestinal function were revealed to be compromised. However, his GI's condition was not considered to be of significance nor related to his complaints according to his previous doctors/ practitioners.

By means of a specialized blood investigation it was shown that the patient had specific antibodies to a number of foodstuffs, in keeping with a type-3 allergy, i.e. the delayed type. Of particular interest were antibodies to milk and milk products, as well as yeast. On questioning, the patient admitted that he consumed these products on a daily basis—they were generally accepted as healthy foods, after all. Yes, perhaps, but not for him, right now!

Excluding those foods to which the patient had developed antibodies caused his symptoms to disappear within a few days; the symptoms did not recur.

To confirm the diagnosis his doctor performed provocation tests. On certain days the patient was asked to ingest these specific foods and we observed the results.

It was found that milk products most frequently led to headache, chronic fatigue and changes of mood.

Yeast caused marked flatulence and abdominal pressure. As the patient had been advised to avoid milk products, a natural source of probiotics (essential beneficial intestinal bacteria) was no longer available. Therefore the patient was prescribed a probiotic supplement.

By altering his diet in this manner, the symptoms nearly disappeared. Without reducing his caloric intake the patient lost a significant amount of weight—which made him very happy—and his other blood indices, like his cholesterol, uric acid, etc. also returned to normal.

However, he still experienced headaches on rare occasions.

It was concluded that there was yet another cause for the patient's headache.

The absence of certain enzymes in the intestines may render it impossible for an individual to disintegrate or detoxify certain substances and this may lead to problems.

On being asked, the patient said he occasionally experienced a headache only after consuming red wine. However, a blood analysis showed that the patient had adequate quantities of the DAO enzyme. His results were just above the necessary threshold value. The histamine content of wine varies, depending on the type of wine and the manufacturing procedure. Unfortunately, the histamine content is not listed on the label. Therefore, the histamine content becomes evident only the next day–depending on whether the individual experiences a headache or not. Not every type of red wine caused a headache in our patient. He was aware of one or the other type which was inevitably followed by a headache the next day. We selected these and he drank his usual amount once as an experiment in conjunction with taking some diamine oxidase, and the another time drinking this wine without taking the DAO enzyme.

Lo and behold–with the DAO, he tolerated the red wine without any difficulties, whereas without the DAO, he experienced a headache the next day. We repeated the test a few times and always achieved the same result. This proved the fact that histamine was one of the causes of the headache experienced by this patient.

For six months the patient has been taking his dose of diamine oxidase before consuming wine and has been having no headaches ever since.

Case report II

The following example again shows how various factors might interact and lead to symptoms in other organs of the body:

A woman, late thirties, complains of regular headache, migraine, most often during menstruation, strong abdominal pain, spasms and constipation.

She does not consume any alcohol.

A change in diet, based on a special blood analysis for type 3 allergies, brought about very little improvement. For obvious reasons it was concluded that the patient had digestive disorders and, possibly, an imbalanced bowel flora as well as a potential histamine intolerance. Particularly the patient's recurrent migraine at menstruation is indicative of this condition. During menstruation, large quantities of histamine are released due to bleeding. This leads to contractions at the uterus and triggers pain. The diamine oxidase level measured in blood was moderately reduced.

A specific stool investigation showed markedly increased clostridia.

Clostridia are bacteria that play a very active role in metabolism. They serve as regular factories of histamine.

In addition to biogenic amines which inhibit diamine oxidase, they release large quantities of histamine which overwhelms the body's detoxification system in addition to the load resulting from the histamine ingested with food. These are also responsible for abdominal cramps and constipation, as well as headaches. Normally these bacteria can be kept under control through a healthy diet. However, when they occur in such high concentrations, antibiotic treatment is often utilized.

Thus, the therapeutic approach was to eliminate the undesired bacterial flora and restore a healthy bowel probiotic population, with a change of dietary habits, and the administration of diamine oxidase, particularly before and during menstruation.

These measures caused the patient's symptoms to subside completely. Thus, it was found that a specific symptom is quite often attributable to more than one cause. In making an accurate diagnosis, the person is frequently confronted with a complex network of inter-related causes, actions and reactions, culminating in a seemingly simple single symptom.

In order to eliminate a problem at its source, at the root cause, it is well-advised to address all components that might be involved, inter-related, and overlap.

Like no other organ system in this regard, the intestines always play a central role in this process. The immune system, neurotransmitter metabolism, hormone generation and metabolism, liver processing and detoxification, as well as kidney function and so many other factors are markedly influenced by the natural and proper functioning of our digestive system.

Therefore, any deficits such as a diamine oxidase deficiency should be balanced and unnecessary strain on the immune system avoided when encountered.

Resources

Histame is the clinically studied DAO preparation that offers hope to the millions of Americans who suffer from food intolerance. Now acknowledged by the U.S. Food and Drug Administration as a new dietary ingredient (NDI), for the first time, the enzyme diamine oxidase (DAO) is available in the United States.

Histame is the first product in the United States that is clinically shown to regulate exogenous histamine levels, elevated by food intake, which can cause food intolerance.

For more information, visit **www.histame.com**

References

F, Ahrens, G, Gabel, B, Garz, JR, Aschenbach: Release and permeation of histamine are affected by diamine oxidase in the pig large intestine. *Inflamm Res* 51 Suppl 1 : S83, 2002

U, Amon, E, Bangha, T, Kuster, A, Menne, IB, Vollrath, BF, Gibbs: Enteral histaminosis: Clinical implications. *Inflamm Res* 48 : 291, 1999

JR, Aschenbach, HG, Schwelberger, F, Ahrens, B, Fürll, G, Gäbel: Histamine inactivation in the colon of pigs in relationship to abundance of catabolic enzymes. *Scand J Gastroenterol* 41 : 712, 2006

TJ, David: Adverse reactions and intolerance to foods. *Br Med Bull* 56 : 34, 2000

L, Maintz, N, Novak: Histamine and histamine intolerance. *Am J Clin Nutr* 85 : 1185, 2007

L, Maintz-Laura, S, Benfadal-Said, JP, Allam-Jean-Pierre, T, Hagemann-Tobias, R, Fimmers-Rolf, N, Novak-Natalija: Evidence for a reduced histamine degradation capacity in a subgroup of patients with atopic eczema. *J Allergy Clin Immunol* 117 : 1106, 2006

C, Ortolani, C, Bruijnzeel-Koomen, U, Bengtsson, C, Bindslev-Jensen, B, Bjorksten, A, Host, M, Ispano, R, Jarish, C, Madsen, K, Nekam, R, Paganelli, LK, Poulsen, B, Wuthrich: Controversial aspects of adverse reactions to food. European Academy of Allergology and Clinical Immunology (EAACI) Reactions to Food Subcommittee. *Allergy* 54 : 27, 1999

C, Ortolani, EA, Pastorello: Food allergies and food intolerances. *Best Pract Res Clin Gastroenterol* 20 : 467, 2006

J, Sattler, D, Hafner, HJ, Klotter, W, Lorenz, , Wagner PK: Food-induced histaminosis as an epidemiological problem: plasma histamine elevation and haemodynamic alterations after oral histamine administration and blockade of diamine oxidase (DAO). *Agents Actions* 23 : 361, 1988

SL, Taylor: Histamine food poisoning: toxicology and clinical aspects. *Crit Rev Toxicol* 17 : 91, 1986

F, Wantke, M, Gotz, , Jarisch R: Histamine-free diet: treatment of choice for histamine-induced food intolerance and supporting treatment for chronic headaches. *Clin Exp Allergy* 23 : 982, 1993

S, Wohrl, W, Hemmer, M, Focke, K, Rappersberger, , Jarisch R: Histamine intolerance-like symptoms in healthy volunteers after oral provocation with liquid histamine. *Allergy Asthma Proc* 25 : 305, 2004

T, Zuberbier, C, Pfrommer, K, Specht, S, Vieths, R, Bastl-Borrmann, M, Worm, BM, Henz: Aromatic components of food as novel eliciting factors of pseudoallergic reactions in chronic urticaria. *J Allergy Clin Immunol* 109 : 343, 2002

About the Author

Marcus Laux, N.D.

Dr. Marcus Laux is a licensed naturopathic physician who received his doctorate from the National College of Naturopathic Medicine (NCNM) in Portland, Oregon. Dr. Laux also received his D. Hom(Med) from the internationally recognized College of Homeopathy.

He has served as an assistant adjunct professor at Emperor's College of Traditional Oriental Medicine and as clinical professor of OB/GYN at NCNM. He is an affiliate faculty member at Bastyr University of Natural Health. For nearly two decades, Dr. Laux maintained a full-time private family practice in Beverly Hills and Malibu.

He has chaired and served on numerous scientific advisory boards for leading natural medicine companies. Dr. Laux was the editor of *Naturally Well Today*, an international monthly newsletter published by Healthy Directions, from 2002-2009.

He is co-author of *User's Guide to the Top 10 Natural Therapies, Natural Woman, Natural Menopause* and other books.

To learn more visit **www.doctormarcuslaux.com.**